FOOD FRONTIERS

The next century will see a tremendous flowering of "functional foods," engineered to promote health in many specific ways. One of the major components of today's—and tomorrow's—functional foods is FOS, the amazing nutrient that sustains and stimulates the helpful microorganisms on which our health depends. Here is the full story of this exciting development in guided nutrition and how it can help you.

ABOUT THE AUTHOR

Robert Crayhon, M.S., C.N. is president of Design for Health, a nutrition and weight-loss clinic in New York City, host of the syndicated radio program "The Voice of Wellness" and author of *Robert Crayhon's Nutrition Made Simple.* He has written for many publications, including the *Townsend Letter for Doctors,* and has appeared on radio and television programs across the country.

THE HEALTH BENEFITS OF FOS

(Fructooligosaccharides)

"FAST FOOD" FOR THE FRIENDLY BACTERIA THAT KEEP US HEALTHY

Robert Crayhon
Foreword by Martin Feldman, M.D.

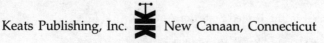

Keats Publishing, Inc.   New Canaan, Connecticut

THE HEALTH BENEFITS OF FOS

Good Health Guides are published by
Keats Publishing, Inc.
27 Pine Street (Box 876)
New Canaan, Connecticut 06840-0876

CONTENTS

FOREWORD

This comprehensive discussion of fructooligsaccharides (FOS) is a milestone in our understanding of naturally occurring food substances that assist the digestive system. This new and exciting carbohydrate targets imbalances in the lower digestive tract, adding one more weapon to the arsenal of natural therapies that can be used to optimize the body's systems.

With the technology available today, FOS can be concentrated in a powder form so that you don't have to eat excessive amounts of the original food to correct digestive imbalances. FOS passes through the system with minimal problems and a low incidence of intolerant or allergic reactions. It is of interest that the digestive system does not break down FOS. Rather, it reaches the lower intestines intact, where it is devoured by the "friendly bacteria" without significantly assisting any of the "unfriendly bacteria." These properties make FOS extremely beneficial in treating a variety of digestive problems.

As a complementary physician with an active practice, I see many patients who suffer from suboptimal digestion. These patients have opted to rebalance their digestive apparatus with natural substances, such as nutrients, herbs, doses of "friendly bacteria," natural anti-parasite and anti-yeast products, acid and pancreatic enzymes and, more recently, FOS.

My job is to direct that process, diagnosing the source of the problems and selecting the most appropriate therapies to treat them. Complementary medicine focuses on optimizing the body so that it functions at its most efficient level, while orthodox medicine focuses primarily on the use of medications in treating a breakdown of functioning. Therefore, complementary physicians view the digestive function in a holistic light, evaluating each component of the system to determine which ones must be rebalanced or repaired. Even though the most severe imbalance may occur in the colon, the intelligent health practitioner must profile the entire system. Natural therapies such as FOS play a major role in that philosophy, and I urge you to put this book to use in your quest for good health.

MARTIN FELDMAN, M.D.
New York, N.Y.

INTRODUCTION

They taste sweet. They're good for you. They occur naturally in foods, and you've been eating them all your life. They're FOS, or fructooligosaccharides. They are a specific food for the beneficial bacteria in your gastrointestinal tract. Because of their ability to stimulate the growth of these critically important bacteria, they are can significantly help you enhance the health of your GI tract and your overall wellness.

The GI tract and the organs that function with it constitute the most important area to focus on in the quest for optimal health. If we do not break down, absorb, and metabolize the nutrients in our food, we are setting the stage for a wide range of ailments. Almost every health disorder is caused or aggravated by a gastrointestinal tract that is functioning suboptimally. Problems as diverse as lack of energy, depression, liver dysfunction and cancer can all be related to an imbalance that begins in the digestive tract.

The saying "death begins in the colon" comes from naturopathic physicians who dominated the medical scene in 19th-century America and were highly aware of the importance of gastrointestinal health. Yet this consciousness has been lost in modern medicine. Few physicians today appreciate the enormous research that has been done showing that a disordered GI tract can cause countless problems. Studies have shown that fiber, beneficial bacteria, and a range of other nutrients are needed on a regular basis to keep the GI tract healthy. Without all of these nutrients, harmful compounds are generated that spread throughout the body. According to researchers such as Jeffrey Bland, Ph.D., a great deal of degenerative disease can be traced to toxicity in the GI tract and liver. It is not far from the truth to say that nearly every ailment begins in or is aggravated by a toxic or malfunctioning digestive tract. While mainstream American medicine has lost sight of the importance of digestive health, the Japanese have not. The Japanese have taught us a lot about healthy eating. The nutrition world has long admired the many beneficial constituents of the Japanese diet: a higher intake of minerals through the many seaweeds they consume, a significant intake of omega-3 fats from their high intake of seafood, and the many benefits of their soy products such as miso, which are high in anticancer compounds. They have also identified the importance of FOS, which they have been using as a food additive since 1983.

Japan leads the world in manufacturing products containing beneficial bacteria such as bifidobacterium. They currently make over 70 foods which contain them.[1] The Japanese government also funds research into the properties of beneficial bacteria, and helps subsidize their placement in food products.

FUNCTIONAL FOODS

Functional foods are foods designed by nutrition scientists to incorporate as many beneficial food factors as possible. Designing a functional food is like assembling a nutritional all-star team with all your favorite food elements to give you benefits that can be superior to those of foods in their natural state. Vitamins, minerals, essential fatty acids, and food concentrates are some of the many constituents that are put into these health-promoting superfoods. The functional food industry is a five billion-dollar industry in Japan, and is growing by leaps and bounds in the U.S. and in Europe. The discovery and production of more beneficial substances like FOS and the increased desire by consumers for foods high in nutritional benefit should place functional foods among the major sellers in the 21st-century supermarket.

Correctly designed, functional foods offer the synergistic effect of a wide range of valuable food components. This effect is more powerful than that achieved by merely consuming one or two valuable nutrients. A well-balanced baseball team is more likely to win than a team with great pitching and poor hitting. Naturally balanced in a variety of health-enhancing constituents, functional foods of the future will also have their "talent" well distributed throughout the team. They will contain a wide variety of nutrients which stimulate detoxifying and immune-enhancing processes. Detoxification and immune enhancement are vital to the functioning of the body, and failure in these areas can lead to many diseases, including liver ailments, heart disease, diabetes and cancer. FOS, as we shall see, is one of the most synergistic and detoxifying players to join the team of functional foods.

Functional foods offer an additional advantage: they are foods that offer the benefits of supplements without the need to take pills or powders. The nutrients are already combined in a food that one eats for pleasure, so functional foods should make getting optimal levels of nutrients in the diet less a medicinal chore than it sometimes seems.

THE MOST IMPORTANT SUPPLEMENTS YOU CAN TAKE

In your gastrointestinal tract, you have approximately three pounds of bacteria. These tenants have great influence over your health. Harmful bacteria, such as *Escherichia coli*, can make you very sick, and are often life-threatening. Beneficial bacteria do the opposite. They promote health, and actually help protect us from a range of toxins. They are also needed for optimal nutrient absorption. In fact, beneficial bacteria and the supplements that support their growth are among the most important supplements you can take for overall health.

Why? Because so many functions of the body are affected by the state of the gastrointestinal tract. Liver health, skin health, blood sugar metabolism, and optimal cholesterol levels depend on a healthy GI tract.

Is FOS a Sweetener or a Fiber?

Both. FOS taste sweet, like sugar, and also cannot be digested by the body, like fiber. FOS are only half as sweet as honey or sugar. Taken in very large amounts, they can cause loose bowels. Yet, with these limitations in mind, FOS may be the "sweetest fiber" ever discovered.

FOS's role as a fiber confers significant benefit. Fiber adds bulk to the stool, and helps the function of the digestive tract in many ways. Optimal fiber intake can
- decrease colon cancer risk
- prevent diverticulosis
- prevent appendicitis
- balance blood sugar
- relieve constipation

FOS, as we have said, are not digestible by the human body. Yet like other fibers, such as apple pectin, FOS are metabolized by bacteria in the GI tract. Their benefits are more wide-reaching than those of any other fiber yet discovered. This is due to FOS's specific ability to promote the growth of beneficial bacteria.

People who live on a diet high in animal products and low in vegetable fiber have fewer beneficial bacteria in their GI tract than those of contrasting habits. Because of this, they are more likely to develop diseases of the intestinal tract.[2] The benefits of fiber may be in large part due to its ability to stimulate the growth of beneficial bacteria such as bifidobacteria. FOS would appear to be a valuable component of any fiber supplement, because it stimulates bifidobacteria growth better than any other fiber. And, unlike other fiber supplements, FOS tastes pleasant.

WHAT ARE FOS?

Fructooligosaccharides are sugars linked together with unique bonds the body can't digest. FOS are sucrose molecules (glucose-fructose disaccharides) to which one, two or three additional fructose molecules have been added. The links that hold these glucose and fructose molecules together are the problem—or the advantage, depending on your point of view. The body contains a great many digestive enzymes. These enzymes' sole task is to "crack the code" that links food molecules together, thus allowing the body to absorb and use them for energy and structural maintenance. Potatoes, rice, and other starches contain molecules of the simple sugar glucose linked together in rows. The body has enzymes that break down these links between the glucose molecules, allowing us to use the glucose for energy. Happily, the body has no enzymes which can digest FOS, letting FOS pass untouched onto the large intestine, where they can feed the beneficial bacteria.

FOS are plural. They are a trio of three different oligosaccharides, working in unison. On the molecular level, they look like the diagram on the next page.

There are other oligosaccharides found in foods as well, but these are the most prominent ones, and the ones found in 95 percent pure FOS products—this degree of purity is considered essential for optimum performance of FOS in the GI tract. These three also are the best promoters of beneficial bacteria in the body.

FOS are a timed-released carbohydrate. They leave the small intestine undigested, and arrive at the large intestine, where the beneficial bacteria, most notably

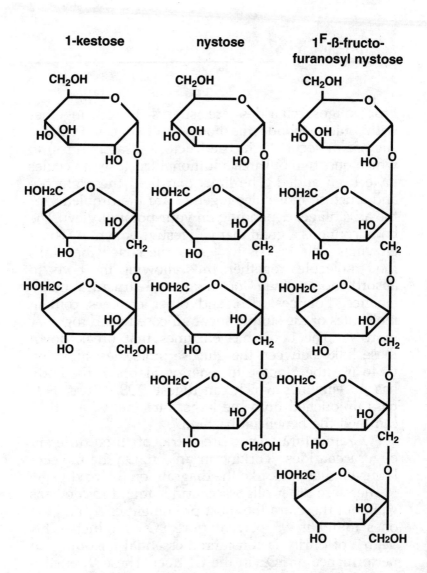

Molecular Structure of Fructooligosaccharides

the bifidobacteria, break the molecule-binding code. Bifidobacteria are able to do what the body and putrefactive bacteria cannot: use FOS for growth and proliferation. When you write a check, you make it out to a particular person , and only that person can cash the check. FOS is the first commercially available dietary supplement with this specificity. It allows you to focus nutritional benefit like a spotlight.

How Many Calories Do FOS Have?

The human body cannot digest FOS, so you might think they have no calories. Yet in their own unique, roundabout way they do. Beneficial bacteria such as bifidobacteria consume FOS. The by-products of this FOS feast are what are called short-chain fatty acids. These fatty acids are absorbed by the walls of the large intestine and used for energy. The body does not consume the FOS directly, but these by-products of bacterial activity. Without bifidobacteria, we would never get any calories from FOS.

By this circuitous route, FOS contribute only approximately 1.5 calories per gram to the body. Digestible carbohydrates give the body 4 calories per gram. Further study is needed to determine the exact caloric content of FOS. However, compared with 9 calories per gram of fat, and 4 calories per gram of protein or carbohydrate, FOS are much lower in calories.

FOS in Foods

The Japanese have over 500 food products that contain FOS. Some of those available are powdered and syrup sweeteners, pastry, candies, pancake syrup, infant formula, cereals, soft drinks, yogurt and tofu. FOS are sold as dietary supplements in powder and liquid form in the United States.

FOS promote the growth of beneficial bacteria. Before we can understand why this is so important and further explore the many benefits of FOS, we have to look at the marvelous function of these beneficial bacteria and the role they play in the body.

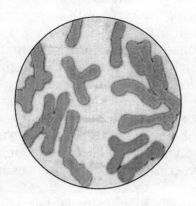

WHAT ARE BENEFICIAL BACTERIA?

"Surely no man would want to live without friends," Aristotle said. Life would not be the same without them. Nutritionally speaking, we need friends, too. The most important nutritional friends make all the difference in our health. They are the beneficial bacteria and the foods which support them. Without them, our health would not be satisfactory, no matter what else we did.

Most physicians do not recognize the key role a healthy gastrointestinal tract plays in maintaining overall health. This is because a healthy GI tract has so many benefits. Sounds paradoxical, but it's true. Physicians are trained to use drugs that have single effects, and are not well equipped to recognize problems or benefits that are multifactorial. They have been trained to mistrust anything that has wide-ranging effects, and believe that something that is said to benefit the entire body is claiming to be a panacea and akin to quackery. For these and other reasons, the importance of a healthy GI tract has been overlooked by modern medicine.

Imagine riding in a car with only three wheels on it, with the fourth wheel base scraping on the ground. Suppose someone told you that if you only added a fourth wheel to your car you could go faster, get better mileage, have better handling, and experience a much smoother ride. Everything about your car and its ride would be helped by this simple addition, and problems you thought were unrelated to this missing wheel would clear up. "Sounds too good to be true," you might say. "How can one thing do all that?"

Anything which, like beneficial bacteria, is essential to the health of every part of the body can have such wide-ranging effects. They are central, irreplaceable parts of everything that happens within us. Without adequate quantities of them, there is hardly any limit to the number of things that can go wrong. But when you understand the central role they play, you'll understand how they can have such a profound influence.

Beneficial bacteria are actually in the minority in the gastrointestinal tract. Beneficial bacteria like bifidobacteria constitute at best a little more than a third of the GI tract's bacterial population. At worst, they may be so low in number as to be undetectable. They are like prison guards supervising the activity of the other bacteria in the GI tract. These other bacteria have varying degrees of disease-causing potential. Beneficial bacteria keep them under control. They prevent a bacterial "riot" that can result in a wide variety of ailments. Sometimes, as after a course of antibiotics, we need to take supplements of beneficial bacteria on a regular basis. Adopting a diet, lifestyle and supplement regime that keeps these bacteria going strong and helps you starve the disease-causing bacteria will help keep the balance of bacteria in your favor.[3]

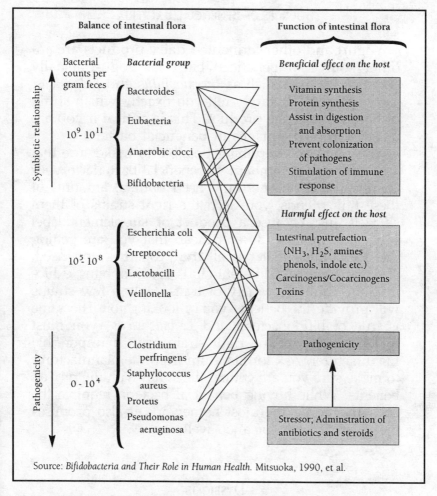

Source: *Bifidobacteria and Their Role in Human Health.* Mitsuoka, 1990, et al.

Types and Effects of Helpful and Harmful Intestinal Bacteria.

The three main kinds of beneficial bacteria are, in order of importance

- *Bifidobacterium*
- *Lactobacillus acidophilus*
- *Lactobacillus bulgaricus*

These supplements are usually found in the refrigerated section of your health food store.

Yogurt and other fermented dairy products are another source of beneficial bacteria. Yogurt usually contains bacteria such as *thermophilus* and *bulgaricus*. Yet yogurt labels rarely tell you exactly which strain of bacteria is in the product. This is critical if you are to enjoy the advantages of beneficial bacteria.

You must do everything possible to make sure that you have a large amount of beneficial bacteria in your GI tract. And you not only need optimal amounts of these tiny friends, you need the right strains of them as well. Just because a product or supplement label says "acidophilus" doesn't mean that you are getting the acidophilus that has all the properties you need. There are over 200 different kinds of acidophilus, exhibiting an immense variety of traits. Only a few strains will provide the benefits you're looking for. The same is true of bifidobacteria and *L. bulgaricus*—you must make sure to get the right strain from a responsible manufacturer. Ask for literature from the manufacturer to make sure you are getting the strain with the proven benefits. While buying beneficial bacteria requires the consumer to do the most homework, it also promises the most rewards for a job well done.

DYSBIOSIS

Dysbiosis is the term scientists use to describe a disordered gastrointestinal situation in which beneficial bacteria are low in number and pathogenic substances have increased dangerously. The following is a list of problems in which dysbiosis is at least a cofactor, if not a primary cause:[4]

- acne
- autoimmune illnesses
- breast cancer
- *Candida albicans* overgrowth

- chronic fatigue syndrome
- colon cancer
- colitis
- depression
- digestive problems
- fatigue
- food allergy and intolerance
- intestinal gas and bloating
- irritable bowel syndrome
- PMS
- rheumatoid arthritis
- schizophrenia

Because food allergy, on our list above, can have such a wide range of symptoms, the list of things

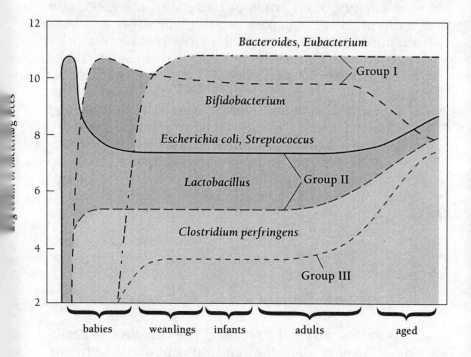

Changes in Fecal Flora with Increased Age.

Source: *Bifidobacteria and their Role in Human Health.* Mitsuoka, 1190, et al.

that can be caused or worsened by dysbiosis is almost limitless. And an excessively large population of harmful bacteria can also stimulate and aggravate many autoimmune diseases. In these ailments the body's dysfunctional immune system turns on the body it is supposed to defend. The list of autoimmune problems in which harmful bacteria and dysbiosis are cofactors is a long one.

WHAT DO BACTERIA EAT?

Bacteria of all kinds can feed on carbohydrates: sugars, and the starches that break down into sugars. Eating sugar or lots of carbohydrates will increase the amount of all kinds of bacteria: some good, and more often the bad. You can think of sugar as a kind of anti-FOS: it encourages the growth of harmful bacteria and parasites. And just as sugar is used to make yeast grow and expand bread dough, too much sugar in the diet can increase the number of yeast organisms such as *Candida albicans*, and lead to intestinal bloating. Candida overgrowth in your GI tract can also cause a lack of ability to concentrate ("spaciness"), depression, and more sugar cravings, to name but a few of the problems. Too many of the pathogenic bacteria such as *Clostridium perfringens* and *E. coli* make a wide variety of compounds that are disease causing.

FRIENDLY BACTERIA AND NUTRIENT ABSORPTION

A gastrointestinal tract filled with unfriendly bacteria will make digestion and absorption of nutrients more difficult. It is fine to supplement your diet with vitamins and other nutrients, but without the right balance of nutrients in the GI tract they will not be absorbed and metabolized optimally. Deficiency states may actually arise.

For example, the amino acid taurine is critical to immune function and cell membrane stability throughout the body. It is excreted in much larger amounts when there are too many unfriendly bacteria in the GI tract. *Candida albicans* in particular may cause a loss of taurine, along with malabsorption of other nutrients, including vitamin B6 and magnesium. Taurine deficiency can lead to a wide range of health problems.[5]

BIFIDOBACTERIA

Though acidophilus is the beneficial bacterium most people are familiar with, bifidobacteria are the most significant microorganisms in the gastrointestinal tracts. There are benefits to be had from acidophilus and bulgaricus, and they should be part of your beneficial bacteria supplement regime. Yet the bifidobacteria are the most important of the beneficial bacteria, and are the ones specifically promoted by FOS. While the benefits of the various types of beneficial bacteria are often similar, we will focus our discussion on bifidobacteria.

Studies show bifidobacteria can:[6]
- Lower cholesterol levels
- Prevent food poisoning and diarrhea
- Produce acids which reduce the pH in the GI tract. The resulting acidic condition makes it difficult for harmful bacteria and other pathogens to live or multiply in the intestinal tract.
- Help the body digest lactose, the sugar found in milk and to a lesser extent in other dairy products. They also increase the digestibility of calcium.
- Increase production of small amounts of natural antibiotics that rid the GI tract of undesirable bacteria

- Make vitamins B1, B2, B6 and B12, niacin and folic acid
- Ease constipation by creating substances that stimulate natural contraction of the muscles of the digestive tract, and by increasing the size of the stool
- Play an important role in preventing autoimmune diseases
- Be a critically important supplement in the treatment of chronic fatigue
- Be important in the treatment of a wide variety of skin disorders, especially acne
- Be useful in the treatment of a wide range of other disorders

One of the negative aspects of a diet high in meat and low in vegetables is that it promotes an increase in harmful bacterial enzymes that produce a great many disease-causing by-products. Skatol, phenol, indole, cresol, amines, ammonia and other harmful substances tend to proliferate on such an unbalanced diet. Too many harmful bacteria can also increase the body load of estrogens, and may increase breast cancer risk. Unfriendly bacteria such as *E. coli* and *C. perfringens* create this wide range of toxins which are harmful to our health. One of the most valuable roles that beneficial bacteria like bifidobacteria play is to exert their focused antibiotic activity and remove harmful bacteria from the GI tract. By making conditions unbearable for these unfriendly bacteria, the friendly bacteria are able to lower the number of these unwanted guests, thereby decreasing the quantity of harmful byproducts produced as well as lessening long-term risk of disease.

NEGATIVE INFLUENCES ON THE GI TRACT

To maintain gastric health, there are many lifestyle factors that need to be avoided as much as possible.

They upset the balance of health in the gastrointestinal tract that can lead to a variety of ailments. Those who knowingly or inadvertently adopt some of the lifestyle factors listed below may very well benefit from supplementing their diets with FOS. Try to avoid:

• Prolonged use of antibiotics, which kill beneficial bacteria. Reducing the quantity of beneficial bacteria in the GI tract allows the harmful ones to overgrow. Follow your physician's recommendations regarding the use of antibiotics. Antibiotics have their place in medicine, and can be lifesaving in acute conditions. They are, however, needlessly overused and abused in chronic conditions for which natural therapies are more effective.

• Antiseptic supplements like goldenseal and grapefruit seed extract can decrease the levels of beneficial bacteria if taken over long periods.[7]

• Sugar consumption in any form and diets high in refined carbohydrates such as white flour are also disruptive to GI bacterial health. Sugar feeds the unfriendly bacteria and encourages an overgrowth of the yeast *Candida albicans*.

BIFIDOGENIC FACTORS

Bifidogenic factors are those foods that help the body increase its levels of beneficial bacteria. These include substances such as N-acetylglucosamine, lactulose found in milk and milk products, and FOS. Lactulose is very expensive, is unavailable except for medical studies, and causes diarrhea. FOS is the best choice. It is inexpensive, convenient, and already used by millions.

BENEFITS OF FOS

Now we know the many benefits of beneficial bacteria. It should now be clear how FOS, a specific food for beneficial bacteria, promotes our health on many levels. FOS increases the number of bifidobacteria and starves the unfriendly bacteria, shifting the balance in our favor.[8]

In order to get the benefit from beneficial bacteria products, one cannot merely take them and assume that they will thrive in the gastrointestinal tract. They may not. Survival of the fittest is the rule in the GI tract, as elsewhere in nature. That's where FOS come in. They selectively feed the beneficial bacteria, and help them multiply and remain strong.

The studies on FOS are very recent, dating from 1983, and more are needed. Yet this small but impressive body of research shows that 95 percent pure FOS promote health in a wide variety of ways.[9] Studies show 95 percent pure FOS can:

• Selectively feed and encourage the growth of beneficial bacteria such as bifidobacterium in the human GI tract. 1 gram per day of FOS has been shown to cause a fivefold increase in bifidobacteria.

• Reduce the growth of unfriendly bacteria and the putrefactive substances they produce in the digestive tract

• Relieve constipation

• Stop antibiotic-associated diarrhea

• Lower blood cholesterol and triglyceride levels

• Improve the taste, texture and health benefits of a wide variety of foods

- Fight the formation of cavities
- Help diabetics lower blood sugar levels
- Provide approximately 1.5 calories per gram, less than one-half the caloric content of other carbohydrates

FOS are a naturally-occurring food component. Humans have always consumed them as part of the everyday diet. So they not only have a wide range of benefits, but are remarkably safe as well. And a little FOS goes a long way towards promoting optimal health.

The Prebiotic FOS Are Not a Replacement for Probiotic Beneficial Bacteria Supplements

FOS increase beneficial bacteria levels, but don't think they are the only supplement you should take to increase the quality and quantity of your good bacteria. FOS are in partnership with beneficial bacteria. They are not meant to replace high-quality beneficial bacteria supplements, but to amplify them. They are much less expensive and more stable than beneficial bacteria—which are comparatively fragile, making their safe arrival in their intestinal lodging sometimes uncertain. This allows them to be added to foods without fear of deterioration. This is an advantage consumers and manufacturers both appreciate, but beneficial bacteria should be a part of a supplementation regime as well as 95 percent pure FOS.

SOURCES OF FOS

FOS are found naturally in many foods. Bananas, onions, garlic, artichokes, barley, tomatoes, rye, honey, asparagus and triticale all contain some FOS. But there are two reasons why you can't rely on food to provide you with optimal amounts of FOS.

There is not enough FOS in foods in the average diet to get an optimal or therapeutically significant dose. As is the case with nutrients like vitamins C and E, optimal doses of FOS cannot entirely come through food. Though bananas, onions, and asparagus have reasonable amounts of FOS, one would have to eat a significant serving of these foods with each meal every day to get a useful dose.

Secondly, most people consume a great deal of refined sugars and flours, and combine this with a diet low in many nutrients. Add stress, alcohol consumption, and the many toxic chemicals in our foods and environment—especially the chlorine in our water—

FOOD	ESTIMATED CONCENTRATION % OF FOS
Garlic	1.0
Honey	1.0
Rye	0.6
Brown Sugar	0.4
Banana	0.3
Onion	0.3
Barley	0.2
Tomato	0.2

FOS Content of Foods

and you make things very difficult for the beneficial bacteria in the GI tract to survive and thrive. Relying on the FOS in food to support the growth of beneficial bacteria in modern, industrialized diets and environments is like planning to survive a hurricane in a tent.

How FOS Are Made

FOS products sold in health food stores are usually fermented by enzymes of the fungus *Aspergillus niger* acting on sucrose to create FOS. The final product is tested for purity with a laboratory test known as high-performance liquid chromatography. The FOS product created by such a process is identical to the FOS found in foods. It allows for optimal FOS intake without all the calories and sugars present in foods such as bananas. These sugars can weaken the benefits of FOS. The manufacturing process also allows for a purity and assured FOS content that cannot be found in food-derived oligosaccharide products.

Other Sources of Oligosaccharides

Oligosaccharides can be derived from other foods, such as soy and Jerusalem artichoke. Soy oligosaccharides do not have the purity and targeted effectiveness of 95 percent pure FOS. And up to 45 percent of soy oligosaccharides consist of sugars such as sucrose, which work to undo the benefits users hope to obtain. Soy oligosaccharides also contain indigestible sugars found in beans that can cause a significant amount of gas in the GI tract.

Jerusalem artichoke flour contains FOS. It also contains a compound known as inulin, which can act as a precursor to FOS.[10]

Inulin is a larger molecule than FOS, and needs to be broken down by the body first into oligosaccharides. This delays any benefit it may confer. Jerusalem artichoke flour is only 21 percent FOS, and is 15 percent sugar. It should therefore not be used in instances of dysbiosis such as Candida overgrowth, in which any sugar consumption will have a negative effect. It also does not dissolve easily in water, and has an unpleasant taste.

There are many preparations of oligosaccharides, from soy to chicory and artichokes and beyond. Experience shows that these products have benefit, and all of them, like FOS, are safe. But the most scientific research has been done on 95 percent pure FOS, which has the best-documented and most positive effects. The advantage of FOS is that it does not have the high level of digestible sugars these other products contain. It is also highest in the most bifidogenic—that is, promoting the growth of bifidobacteria—types of the oligosaccharides.

FOS Products

You can get 95 percent pure FOS in syrup or powder form. Both are equally beneficial. The only way to know what variety of FOS you are getting, whether powder or syrup, is to contact the manufacturer to see if 95 percent purity is guaranteed. In the future, it is to be expected that responsible manufacturers will tell you their product is at least 95 percent pure FOS on the product label. A very sweet taste is a sign you are not buying 95 percent pure FOS; the product should be only mildly sweet.

CLINICAL APPLICATIONS

With their functions so intertwined, it can be hard to separate the benefits of bifidobacteria from those of FOS. There must be bifidobacteria present in the gastrointestinal tract for FOS to be helpful. FOS increases the activity of the bifidobacteria, but taking bifidobacteria at the same time will boost the benefit of FOS.

BLOOD PRESSURE

Sugar is a food that is not recommended for those with high blood pressure. There is some evidence suggesting that sugar upsets the metabolism of the hormone insulin, and through this mechanism may raise blood pressure. Sugar also depletes the body of minerals that are needed to keep blood pressure in balance.

FOS will do none of these things, and actually has been shown to lower blood pressure slightly in hypertensives. One study showed that 11.5 grams per day of FOS lowered diastolic blood pressure an average of 6 mmHg (millimeters of mercury, the standard measurement of blood pressure—6 mmHg represents about 9 percent of normal diastolic blood pressure) in 46 patients. Many studies show that FOS can lower blood pressure.[11]

Candida Albicans

Taking supplements of beneficial bacteria is a good idea. Yet we need to do everything we can to encourage that these beneficial strains survive in our GI tract. In cases of *Candida albicans* overgrowth and other states of dysbiosis, taking supplements of bifidobacteria and the other beneficial bacteria alone is often not enough. We need to do everything we can to make sure that the beneficial bacteria survive and grow over the long term. This will reduce the amount of Candida in the body. FOS play a key role in helping do this, and helping ensure—like a clamp on a wood joint that has just been glued together—that the supplements of beneficial bacteria will take. It is also important to make sure that you are getting 95 percent FOS, and that it is not diluted with other non-FOS sugars that can feed the Candida and thus defeat the benefit of FOS.

Diabetes and FOS

Can there be a healthy sweetener for diabetics? It is worth considering FOS for the role of an important supplemental food and sweetening agents for those with blood sugar disorders of all kinds. FOS have a sweet taste, something that diabetics are usually not encouraged to enjoy. FOS have a range of benefits for diabetics. Diabetics who were given 8 grams of FOS for 14 days showed a significant decrease in both fasting blood glucose levels and total cholesterol levels.

There are various speculations as to how FOS help diabetics, but the mechanism has not been fully elucidated. FOS may help diabetics by binding in a fiberlike fashion to carbohydrates and fats. FOS may also help diabetics by altering the bowel flora toward a more favorable population. This reduces the production of toxic compounds that can harm the liver. This in turn may reduce the absorption of carbohydrates and fats, causing cholesterol and blood sugar levels to decline. Human studies have shown that FOS acts mainly to lower the LDL cholesterol, the potentially "harmful" type. FOS also raises levels of beneficial HDL cholesterol. These benefits have also been demonstrated in animal studies.[12]

Diabetics also often suffer from constipation and impaired contraction of the gallbladder. Both of these problems are thought to be caused by nerve damage to the autonomic nervous system, which often occurs as a side effect of diabetes. Daily doses of 8 to 10 grams of FOS were given to 13 diabetic patients for four weeks. Nine of the patients experienced relief from constipation, and six showed improved contraction of the gallbladder. There was also a significant increase in the population of bifidobacteria in the intestinal flora of these patients. There was also a reduction in the quantity of pathogenic bacteria such as Clostridium. This shift in bowel flora is thought to be the cause of the improved intestinal function, for the FOS had no effect on the diabetic neurosis in these patients.[13]

Overgrowth of *E. coli* in the intestinal tract may also dispose one to a diabetic condition, and may worsen diabetes. This pathogen can produce a substance very similar to insulin that can block the functioning of the body's own insulin.

FOS may well be the sweetener of choice for diabetics. While it has only half the sweetness of most other sweeteners, its many benefits without any downside may persuade diabetics to give up some of the sweetness of the harmful sugars to gain the significant advantages of FOS. But, in this as in other instances, 95 percent pure FOS is needed for the desired effect.

FOS have been shown in animal and human studies to lower triglyceride and cholesterol levels. They have also been shown to increase levels of HDL cholesterol, the "protective" cholesterol, whose benefits in preventing heart disease are well documented. In fact, many researchers feel that the ratio of total cholesterol to HDL is more important than the total cholesterol number alone. There are few foods that can help lower total cholesterol and raise HDL cholesterol, and studies indicate FOS can do both.[11]

One of the offending foods that causes cholesterol and triglyceride to go up is sugar, and another is refined carbohydrates like white flour. Reducing intake of these junk foods has helped many lower their cholesterol levels, especially when combined with supplements of chromium picolinate, no-flush niacin (inositol hexanicotinate) and aged garlic extract. Yet persons on a cholesterol-lowering program often insist on sugar as a sweetener, sabotaging their other nutritional efforts. FOS seems to be a good alternative.

It is thought that FOS are able to lower cholesterol levels by decreasing the amount of cholesterol made in the liver. Many of the drugs now used to lower cholesterol block the function of an enzyme called HMG-CoA reductase, which the liver requires in order to make cholesterol. Blocking the function of HMG-CoA reductase lowers cholesterol. The trouble with these medications is their many undesirable side effects. Lovastatin is one of the best-known HMG-CoA reductase inhibitor medications. Its side effects include muscle damage, cramps, liver damage, gastrointestinal problems and kidney failure.[15] Clofibrate, another lipid-lowering medication, was studied by the World Health Organization and found to lead to a 44 percent increased mortality rate in the 5,000 patients sampled.[15]

FOS appear to reduce the activity of the HMG-CoA reductase and subsequent cholesterol formation without these dangerous side effects. It appears to work like this: when bifidobacteria consume FOS, they produce short chain fatty acids (SCFA) which interrupt the activity of HMG-CoA, thus lowering cholesterol levels.

KIDNEY FAILURE

FOS have been studied in those with chronic renal failure, and have been found to be safe and effective in increasing their beneficial bacterial populations. Nine patients took 6 grams of FOS for 12 months. Amounts of putrefactive substances decreased, as did cholesterol and triglyceride levels. Constipation was relieved. There were no side effects.[16]

Animal studies have also pointed to another benefit of FOS for kidney failure patients. FOS have been found to decrease the amount of nitrogen and urea excretion by 20 to 30 percent. This reduces the stress on the kidney, and could be of significant benefit to those with renal failure. Further human studies are needed.[17]

LIVER FUNCTION

In my practice I have found that FOS are of benefit to those with liver ailments. The liver has innumerable functions, and optimal health requires an optimally functioning liver. When there are toxic substances being produced in the gastrointestinal tract by unfriendly bacteria, the liver has to deal with these substances. An overload of these byproducts can harm our liver and reduce its ability to maintain optimal health. Just as too much alcohol stresses the liver and causes disease, too much of any toxins can cause liver dysfunction.

Both bifidobacteria and FOS can benefit the liver by helping to put out the fire at its source. Decreasing the number of pathogenic substances and free radicals produced in our digestive tract substantially lightens the liver's detoxifying load, so that it can keep up with its other duties in maintaining health. Since there are innumerable ailments related to toxicity resulting from an overloaded liver, FOS and bifidobacteria may have a wide range of applications in treating and preventing a considerable variety of these health problems.

FOS AND AGING

As we age, we have less of the beneficial bacteria in our GI tract. Digestive complaints are very common in older people, and a decreased amount of beneficial bacteria may be one of the reasons. FOS appears to be useful in helping older individuals maintain their digestive health and in avoiding ailments of the digestive tract, including constipation, which afflicts a large percentage of older Americans. FOS have been studied in seniors, and have been found to increase the amount of beneficial bacteria by more than 50 percent in as little as a week of supplementation.[18]

CAN FOS HELP US LIVE LONGER?

There are many harmful effects created by the wrong kind of bacteria in our gastrointestinal tract. Mice that live in a germ-free environment live 50 percent longer than normal. This may be due to the decreased amount of free radicals in their system due to the lack of any detrimental bacteria in their GI tracts.

One of the ways in which the human body ages is by the damage inflicted by free radicals. Free radicals are highly unstable compounds that damage cell membranes and other structures in the body. Free radical-caused damage has been implicated in a broad range of diseases, including heart disease, cancer, arthritis and Alzheimer's disease.

The largest site of free radical formation in the body is the large intestine,[19] and FOS help limit the amount of free radicals produced in the colon. By so doing, they may help us avoid a great many diseases throughout the body.

WHAT FOS INTAKE IS OPTIMAL?

More research is needed for us to know exactly how much FOS is needed for optimum health. Small amounts, such as one gram per day, or about ¼ teaspoon, seem to be the minimal effective dose. The effects of FOS are cumulative. As is true of many other nutrients, the real benefit of FOS comes with regular consumption over a long period of time, not occasional intake. Taking small amounts over the long term is the best way to derive benefit from FOS.

This is why the growing development of functional foods movement is promising. Putting FOS in a wide variety of foods provides the benefits of regular FOS consumption without the inconvenience of taking it as a supplement.

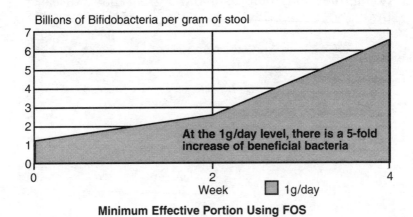

Minimum Effective Portion Using FOS

COOKING WITH FOS

Can FOS be used in place of sugar in recipes? To some degree. FOS are sweet, but they are only half as sweet as sugar, so you need to use more FOS to get the same degree of sweetness. Yet large amounts of FOS can cause loose bowels in some people. This will vary from person to person. This factor, plus the high amounts needed to match the sweetness of honey or sugar, makes it hard to use them as a complete replacement for sugar. Yet FOS can be used as a partial replacement for sugar in any recipe. Experiment and see which amount suits you best.

What makes FOS wonderful is what makes them tricky. Because they are not absorbed, they can loosen the bowels if taken in large amounts. The body cannot absorb FOS and ushers them out quickly if there is too much. Yet many have found that if they increase their dose of FOS gradually, they can tolerate up to a teaspoon—four times the initial minimum dose—at a time. It is advisable to work up to that dose slowly, over a period of a week or so.

FOS can, however, be added in small amounts to many recipes to enhance their nutritional benefit. Try adding small amounts of FOS syrup to teas and drinks, and use either the powder or syrup in small amounts in baked goods of all kinds. Taste tests show that people prefer yogurt with the slightly increased sweetness FOS can offer. FOS can also increase the creaminess and firm texture of products such as yogurt.

Those who love baking will be happy to know that FOS are very good at adding moisture to food. This means FOS are not only healthier than sugar, for they are not absorbed by the body, but that they hold onto moisture, which is important in light of the increasing amount of fat-free cooking being done. Look for FOS in an increasing number of fat-free items in your natural foods store. FOS do not require refrigeration. Do not put them in a cold or moist environment. The moist environment of the refrigerator may cake the powder, and the syrup can begin to crystallize at colder temperatures. If your FOS syrup has crystallized slightly, this is perfectly normal, and occurs in colder climates. The crystals will disappear upon slight heating.

SAFETY

Animal studies show that FOS do not promote cancer, nor are they toxic in any way, even in large doses.[20] FOS have not been found to have any adverse effects on the DNA, the blueprint of life in our cells. They are not mutagenic or genotoxic in any way. Since FOS are naturally found in foods such as bananas, onions, garlic and tomatoes, which have been consumed since prehistoric times, it would seem that they have already established a safe place in our diet.

As we have seen, the only noted undesirable side effect of large doses of FOS is loose bowels. Yet one needs to consume over 40 grams to get loose bowels from FOS. This is a very large dose. People do differ in their sensitivity to indigestible oligosaccharides. And remember: FOS and the beneficial bacteria they promote can actually help stop diarrhea. As with every nutrient, there is an optimal intake of FOS, and we need to stay within that range. More studies are needed to pinpoint the optimal dose, which will probably vary from person to person. Almost everyone finds that increasing amounts slowly up to one tablespoon per day will not have any bowel-loosening effects.

Another way which FOS can cause a temporary and harmless loosening of bowels is when they help foster a die-off of unfriendly bacteria. FOS increase the number of bifidobacteria, and bifidobacteria can effectively kill many pathogenic organisms, including overgrowths of *Candida albicans*. This die-off is quite desirable, and is in fact one of the benefits of FOS.

In either case, though, one can simply eat less FOS and the bowel looseness will stop.

Some also notice an increase in gas with FOS. This is the result of carbon dioxide being given off by the body as a by-product of the consumption of short-chain fatty acids. Short-chain fatty acids, you will remember, are created by the beneficial bacteria from their FOS feast.[18] Again, the solution is to start with small amounts of FOS and increase dosage gradually. FOS have been repeatedly shown to suppress the proliferation of harmful bacteria and their undesirable by-products. No studies have ever shown an increase in harmful bacteria due to FOS, but further research is needed in this area.

Ideally, one should take supplements of bifidobacterium and other beneficial bacteria when beginning to use FOS. Studies have shown that persons whose health is compromised can have almost undetectably low levels of bifidobacteria. Starting with probiotic supplements in addition to the prebiotic FOS, is best, especially for those who are ill or have any kind of gastrointestinal problems.

SUMMARY

FOS are a prebiotic dietary supplement with a great number of health benefits. We are only beginning to learn of their positive influence on health. We can expect to see them increasingly used in the expanding group of functional foods that are designed to do something unfortunately unknown in the history of nutrition: promote optimal health throughout the population through the everyday foods we consume.

More studies are needed for us to know the full range of the benefits of FOS. They are safe, and have been consumed for as long as we have eaten the countless plant foods they are found in. We are only beginning to understand their benefits.

WHAT SHOULD FUTURE STUDIES OF FOS CONSIDER?

In the future, there will hopefully be studies that will let us know whether FOS will help with a variety of gastrointestinal disorders, including ulcers, hiatus hernia, Crohn's disease, ulcerative colitis and irritable bowel syndrome. In my nutrition practice, I have found FOS a useful tool in these conditions and all problems involving the digestive tract. Clinical studies are needed to establish their benefit in these ailments with scientific certainty.

Another area where FOS may be found to be of benefit relates to the volatile fatty acids they generate. One of these, butyric acid, is currently being studied in clinical trails as an anticancer drug. FOS's ability to increase levels of butyric acid deserves further study.

One of the remarkable things about FOS is that there has yet to be a study published that failed to show some therapeutic benefit. Even vitamins and minerals will fail to show benefits in some studies, depending on what results are being sought. Yet FOS have demonstrated their value, and will presumably continue to do so. This is not surprising. Anything that so significantly affects the health of the gastrointestinal tract, the area most central to human health, is bound to prove increasingly valuable as more studies are done.

GLOSSARY

Acidophilus A family of 200 different beneficial bacteria that reside primarily in the small intestine.

Bifidobacterium A genus of bacteria that reside primarily in the large intestine. Common forms include *Bifidobacterium infantis, B. adolescentis, B. bifidum, B. breve* and *B. longum.*

Clostridium perfringens An unfriendly bacterium commonly found in the human gastrointestinal tract.

Dysbiosis An unhealthy balance of bacteria in the GI tract, involving an overgrowth of unhealthy organisms, including *Candida albicans* and a variety of other harmful bacteria and parasites.

E. coli *Escherichia coli,* a common bacterium which lives in the human gastrointestinal tract. *E. coli* makes many by-products which are unhealthy for the GI tract. Keeping *E. coli* populations low is desirable.

FOS Fructooligosaccharides, a mixture of three sugars linked together to form three oligosaccharides. These three oligosaccharides are made from fructose and glucose linked together.

Fructose A simple sugar found in fruits and vegetables. Fructose is digestible by the body but FOS are not.

Functional foods Manmade foods designed to promote health. Some functional foods may also be designed to address specific health problems that afflict portions of the population. They can contain vitamins, minerals, essential fatty acids, beneficial bacteria, FOS, botanical extracts and other health-promoting factors.

Jerusalem artichoke flour The food highest in natural FOS content. It is only 21 percent FOS, however, and does not provide the benefit level of 95 percent FOS supplements.

Inulin A polysaccharide found in artichoke flour that the body can break down into beneficial oligosaccharides.

Neosugar Another name used for 95 percent pure FOS.

Oligosaccharides Sugars that are at least three molecules long, though not as long as the polysaccharides found in starch.

Prebiotics Substances that are not digestible by the human system but are digestible by bifidobacteria.

Probiotics The live bacterial supplements used to support the beneficial bacterial population of the gastrointestinal tract.

Putrefactive products Substances such as indole, skatol, cresol, phenol, amines and ammonia which are made by unfriendly bacteria in the gastrointestinal tract. These substances are believed to cause many of the diseases of the GI tract. This is why keeping gastrointestinal populations of unfriendly bacteria under control is important. FOS and beneficial bacteria decrease the amount of the putrefactive products found in the GI tract.

Short chain fatty acids (SCFAs) Compounds produced by beneficial bacteria as a result of consuming fibers like FOS. SCFAs are responsible for many of the desirable side effects of FOS, including reduction in putrefactive substances and cholesterol lowering. They also lower the pH of the gastrointestinal tract, which may be important for colon cancer prevention.

REFERENCES

1 McKellar, R. C., Yaguchi, M., Molder, H.W., "Bifidobacteria and Bifidogenic Factors, *Canadian Institute of Food Science and Technology Journal* 23 (1): 29-41 (1990).
2 Benno, Y. et al., "Comparison of Fecal Microflora of Elderly Persons in Rural and Urban Areas of Japan," *Applied Environmental Microbiology* 55: 1100-1105 (1989).
3 Mitsuoka, T., "Bifidobacteria and Their Role in Human Health," *Journal of Industrial Microbiology*, 6: 263-268 (1990).
4 Gotteshall, E., *Breaking the Vicious Circle*, Kirkton Press, Ontario, 1994.
5 Bradford, Robert and Allen, Henry, *Taurine in Health and Disease*, Bradford Research Institute, Chula Vista, Cal., 1988, p. 10.
6 Rasic, J. L. and Kurman, J., *Bifidobacteria and Their Role*, Birkhauser Verlag, Boston, 1983
7 Willard, Terry, *Textbook of Modern Herbology*, Progressive Publishing, Calgary, 1993, p. 104.
8 Hidaka, H. et al., "Effects of Fructooligosaccharides on Intestinal Flora and Human Health," *Bifidobacteria Microflora* 5 (1): 37-50 (1986).
9 Toshiaki Kono, "Fructooligosaccharides," in *Oligosaccharides, Production, Properties, and Applications*, Teruo Nakakuki, ed., Gordon and Breach, Tokyo, 1993, 50-78.
10 GrootWassink, J., Fleming, S., "Non-specific B-fructofuranosidase (inulinase) from Kluyveromyces fragilis: Batch and Continuous Fermentation, Simple Recovery Method and Some Industrial Properties," *Enzyme Microb Technol* 2: 45-53 (1980).
11 Hidaka, H. et al., "Proliferation of Bifidobacteria by Oligosaccharides and Their Useful Effect on Human Health," *Bifidobacteria Microflora* 10(1), 65-79 (1991).

12 Yamashita, K. et al., "Effects of Fructo-oligosaccharides on Blood Glucose and Serum Lipids in Diabetic Subjects," *Nutrition Research* 4: 961-966 (1984).

13 Sano, T., "Effects of Neosugar on Constipation, Intestinal Microflora and Gallbladder Contraction in Diabetes," *Proceedings of the Third Neosugar Conference,* Tokyo (1986).

14 London, S. et al., "Cholesterol-lowering Agent Myopathy (CLAM)," *Neurology* 41: 1159-1160 (1991).

15 "The National Cholesterol Education Program Expert Panel. Report on Detection, Evaluation, and Treatment of High Blood Cholesterol in Adults," *Archives of Internal Medicine* 148: 36-69 (1988).

16 Takahashi, Y., "Effects of Neosugar in the Chronic Renal Failure Patient," *Proceedings of the Third Neosugar Conference,* (Summary) Tokyo, 1986.

17 Younes, H. et al., "Fermentable Fibers or Oligosaccharides Reduce Urinary Nitrogen Excretion by Increasing Urea Disposal in the Rat Cecum," *Journal of Nutrition* 125 (4): 1010-1016 (1995).

18 Mitsuoka, T. et al., "Effect of Fructooligosaccharides on Intestinal Microflora," *Die Nahrung* 31: 5-6 (1987).

19 Babbs, C.F., "Free Radicals and the Etiology of Colon Cancer," *Free Rad Biol Med* 8 (2): 191-200 (1990).

20 Inoue, H., "Long-term Safety of Neosugar in the Rat," Summary from *The Proceedings of the 3rd Neosugar Conference,* Tokyo, 1986.